ATKINS DIET COOKBOOK

The Complete Meal Plan for a Healthy Atkins Lifestyle

EMILIA ROBERTS

Contents

Disclaimer Notice	v
Introduction	vii
1. All About The Atkins Diet	1
2. Phase One Shopping List & Meal Plan	10
3. Phase One Recipes	16
4. Phase Two Shopping List & Meal Plan	39
5. Phase Two Recipes	45
6. Phase Three Shopping List & Meal Plan	67
7. Phase Three Recipes	72
Afterword	97

Disclaimer Notice

Please note the information contained within this document is for educational and entertainment purposes only. Every attempt has been made to provide accurate, up to date and reliable complete information. No warranties of any kind are expressed or implied. Readers acknowledge that the author is not engaging in the rendering of legal, financial, medical or professional advice. The content of this book has been derived from various sources. Please consult a licensed professional before attempting any techniques outlined in this book.

By reading this document, the reader agrees that under no circumstances is the author responsible for any losses, direct or indirect, which are incurred as a result of the use of information contained within this document, including, but not limited to, errors, omissions or inaccuracies.

The trademarks that are used are without any consent, and

the publication of the trademark is without permissions or backing by the trademark owner. All trademarks and brands within this book are for clarifying purposes only and are the owned by the owners themselves, not affiliated with this document.

Introduction

Are you tired of trying diets and failing? Are you desperate to lose weight and become healthier, but it never seems to happen?

Perhaps you're simply on the wrong diet!

If you have read anything about lifestyle and weight loss over the last few years you will no doubt have heard about the Atkins Diet. This is a diet which has had its fair share of controversy, but it is also proven to be ultra-effective, all at the same time.

It's also worth mentioning that the diet has undergone some major changes since it was first invented, and it is now much easier to follow, much more satisfying, and much more sustainable.

What is the Atkins Diet?

Basically, the Atkins Diet is a low carbohydrate plan, but it's

Introduction

quite wrong to call it a 'diet'; once you are on the Atkins, you're on it for life. This isn't ultra-restrictive because there are several phases that you work through, with the most restrictive one being step one. By the time, you reach the final step, you are on a maintenance phase, and this means your lifestyle plan which is easy to follow, fills you up, gives you plentiful vitamins and minerals, and also helps you maintain a healthy diet.

In our first chapter we will explain in more detail what happens to your body when you are on the Atkins Diet, but for now you simply need to realize that you are going to be switching what your body burns for fuel. By fuel we mean how it generates energy to enable your body to move, your organs to function, and generally for your body to do what it needs to do. Normally we burn carbohydrates for fuel, and this is the factory setting that your body comes in, e.g. your default setting; now, when you on a low carbohydrate diet, your body is forced to rethink its fuel burning efforts because carbs are in short supply. By doing this, you are forcing your body into a natural state called ketosis, and this flicks the switch to change from burning carbs to burning fat.

Ketosis is not dangerous, and again we will talk about this in our next chapter. What you need to know at this point is that by embarking on a low carbohydrate diet you will lose weight much faster, you will have more energy, and you will basically be healthier overall, provided you stick to the phases as they go, one by one.

So, are you ready to learn more about the Atkins Diet? It's important to keep an open mind at this stage because you will no doubt have negative connotations from the press ringing in your ears. The important thing to remember? The Atkins Diet is safe, it is healthy, and provided you stick to it properly, it is a very sustainable way to lose weight, maintain it and become healthier overall.

So, without further ado, let's learn more about the Atkins Diet, look at a few meal plans to get you started, and help you find some delicious recipes you can try at home.

1

All About The Atkins Diet

This book is designed to give you an introduction to the Atkins Diet, and then help you get started with a few meal plans for each phase. Before we get onto that, let's discuss how to follow the diet in the first place.

The Atkins Diet is a low carbohydrate diet which takes you through four phases to completion. The end phase is the phase you will remain in for the rest of your life. It's important to realize that there is nothing 'faddy' about the Atkins Diet, and once you are on it, you need to view it as a lifestyle change.

The phases of the Atkins Diet are:

- Phase 1 – Introduction phase
- Phase 2 – Food induction phase
- Phase 3 – Ongoing weight loss phase
- Phase 4 – Maintenance phase

By cutting down the amount of carbs you consume per day, you are forcing your body into a naturally occurring state, called ketosis.

What is Ketosis

Ketosis is vital for the Atkins Diet to work, but it's important to realize that there is nothing unsafe about it. Ketosis occurs when you limit the amount of carbs you consume, and your body suddenly wonders what is happening. This is normal because you are shocking your system in some ways, and it is thinking (falsely) that it is going to starve. When your body thinks it is going to starve, it starts to produce something called ketones, and whilst these are totally safe, some people panic about the whole subject.

Put simply, ketosis is something your body does naturally, and it is really a trick because you are of course not going to starve, you are simply eating in a different way. These ketones are not going to harm you, however for the first phase of the diet, you may find that you experience a few side effects. These side effects will pass quickly, but it is really a case of hanging on in there until they pass.

Ketosis effects are like anything in life; it is a period of time where you need to adjust, and once you have adjusted life will become infinitely easier.

The main side effects which are known to affect the first phase of the Atkins Diet, by forcing your body into ketosis, are:

- Going to the toilet to pee quite frequently

- Dizziness
- Lethargy
- Headaches
- Initial cravings
- Muscle cramps
- Sleep disruption

These effects are all totally normal, and should pass within a couple of weeks to a month. If, however, you notice that they are prolonged or severe, you should seek medical help immediately. If you have any present medical conditions, you should discuss with your doctor regarding your suitability for the Atkins Diet before you start.

The Benefits of the Atkins Diet

We have talked about the potential side effects, but what are the benefits? Of course there are major benefits, otherwise so many people wouldn't attempt the diet in the first place!

The main benefit of the Atkins Diet is dramatic weight loss, but there are other happy effects besides this:

- **Weight loss is guaranteed** – It is impossible to go follow the Atkins Diet properly and not lose weight!
- **Acne symptoms are reduced** – There has been a lot of evidence to show that the Atkins Diet can help clear up acne symptoms and outbreaks.
- **You can easily find a weight which is suitable for you and maintain it easily** – The Atkins Diet final phase is about maintenance, and

you will easily be able to find out your body's 'happy weight'. This means a weight which you can maintain without too much trouble.

- **You will learn about healthy food choices** – Because you are focused on what you are eating much more than you will have been before, you are going to be much more able to make the right choices, which benefit your overall health and wellbeing.
- **You will lose fat from the areas that you actually want to lose it from** – A low carb diet targets visceral fat, which is basically the stuff that sits there all wobbly and annoying. General low calorie diets don't target this type of fat, they target the subcutaneous fat instead, and that is why you often don't lose weight from the areas you want to lose it from with regular diets.
- **Lower changes of diabetes in the future** – There is a lot of evidence to suggest that by following the Atkins Diet properly, you will have less change of developing diabetes. This is because when you limit the amount of carbs you consume, you are lowering your insulin levels too. This is linked to diabetes development, so lower levels is good news for preventions.
- **A boost for your good cholesterol** – Bad cholesterol, aka LDL, needs to be reduced if you are going to have good heart health. On the other hand, HDL, aka good cholesterol, is increased when you are on the Atkins Diet. HDL carries cholesterol out of the body, whereas LDL actually

carries it around the body from the liver. The Atkins boosts HDL.
- **Less chance of a stroke, lower blood pressure and increased heart health** – This is probably to do with the LDL boost and the fact that the Atkins Diet is known to maintain lower blood pressure. Your risk of having a stroke or developing heart disease is therefore slashed.
- **Increased sleep quality** – After the first phase of the diet is over you will notice that your sleep pattern is much more regular and your sleep is of a higher quality.
- **More energy** – Again, after the first phase you will notice a huge boost in your energy and productivity levels, which is great news when you have a long to do list!
- **Goodbye to cravings** – At first you are going to crave things because your body is wondering what is going on, but after that you will notice that cravings are a thing of the past. This is because higher fat foods, which the Atkins Diet encourages, are much more satisfying and will keep you fuller for longer.

As you can see, by following the Atkins Diet, you have a lot to gain! The first phase is going to be hard at first, but if you can hang on in there and grit your teeth through the initial cravings and tiredness, you will see a huge silver lining at the end of it.

The Atkins Diet Phases

We mentioned that the Atkins Diet is made up of four phases, so let's check them out one by one to increase your understanding.

Phase 1 – Introduction Phase

This is the hardest phase because you are beginning your Atkins Diet and your body needs time to adjust. This is also the most restrictive phase, but it doesn't last for long!

Important points of phase one include:

- Consume 20g of net carbs per day only
- Do not consume less than 18g of net carbs
- Do not consume more than 22g of net carbs
- This phase will last for a minimum of two weeks
- This phase should last until you are 15lb away from achieving your goal weight
- If you want to, you can stay in this phase longer than 2 weeks for extra weight loss, but you should be careful of pushing your body too far, too fast
- Eat 4-6oz of protein every single day
- Remember to eat fat because this is what you need to teach your body to burn
- Have three solid meals per day
- You can have snacks, but only two per day, in-between meals
- Add salt to your meals, to avoid mineral loss problems
- Drink plenty of water to help speed up weight loss and keep your body hydrated

Phase 2 – Food Induction Phase

In phase one you will start to introduce different foods into your diet, and that means you are allowed a slightly higher net carb amount per day. Despite that, it's important to remember to keep your protein allowance on par, for overall health.

Important points in phase two include:

- Consume 25g of net carbs per day only
- Phase two can begin two weeks after commencing the diet, i.e. you follow phase one for two weeks and then begin phase two. This will give you a slowly and steady weight loss
- You should keep an eye on your weight during this phase, to ensure that you are not eating too much in the way of carbs. You should weigh yourself weekly and keep an eye on the numbers
- Stay in phase two until you are around 10lb in weight away from your end goal
- Side effects in this phase should be non-existent, or at least massively improved

Phase 3 – Ongoing Weight Loss Phase

Phase three is the point at which you will achieve your goal and move onto maintaining it. In this phase you again increase the amount of net carbs you can consume per day, and you should also note that weight loss is not going to be as fast in this phase as in the first and second phases.

Important points in phase three include:

- You should consume 35g of net carbs per day
- If you notice that your weight is gaining slightly or staying put, drop your carb intake down to 30g of net carbs per day, and then up it slowly to 35g again a short time later
- Remain in phase three until you have reached your goal and also until it has stayed static for a month without fluctuating too much
- Phase three helps you understand your body's carb tolerance, without gaining weight

Phase 4 – Maintenance Phase

Phase four is when you have reached your goal and you are now ready to maintain it for the rest of your life. Well done! You've done a lot of hard work and the results have paid off by this point.

The biggest mistake many people make at this point is thinking that the hard work is over and that they can now eat whatever they want – this is only going to mean that the scales creep up rather dramatically over time.

Important points in phase four include:

- Phase four goes on for the rest of your life, and this is now your lifestyle plan
- You will now know how much carb level is right for your body without increasing your weight
- If you find that your weight begins to creep up slightly you can reduce your carb level in 5g increments and then increase it up again in 5g

increments until everything evens itself out – never drop below the phase 1 amount
- Phase four is about moderation, so whilst you can incorporate the odd treat, remember the word MODERATION!

You now know everything you need to know about following the Atkins Diet, and its now time to get practical and show a few meal plan examples, as well as recipes to help you become creative in the kitchen!

2

Phase One Shopping List & Meal Plan

We have mentioned that phase one is the hardest and most restrictive part of the Atkins Diet, but everything has to start somewhere!

This is a week-long meal plan and shopping list, to get you kick-started weight loss and health success.

Shopping List for One Week of Phase One

- Extra virgin olive oil
- Onions
- Roasted bell peppers
- Tomatoes
- Basil
- Cayenne pepper
- Eggs

- Unsalted butter
- Cooked fresh ham
- Garlic
- Sweet red peppers
- Sweet green peppers
- Canola vegetable oil
- Mozzarella cheese
- Whole grain soy flour
- Sweetener (sugar substitute)
- Cinnamon
- Baking powder
- Baking soda
- Buttermilk
- Sugar free vanilla syrup
- Canola cooking spray
- Turkey breakfast sausage
- Monterey Jack cheese
- Cheddar cheese
- Heavy cream
- Parmesan cheese
- Chocolate whey protein
- Sugar free hazelnut syrup
- Asparagus
- Sun-dried tomatoes
- Balsamic vinegar
- Red wine vinegar
- Scallions/spring onion
- Ground veal
- Ground beef
- Ground pork
- Real mayonnaise

- Dijon mustard
- Celery
- Bratwurst
- Canned sauerkraut
- Brussels Sprouts
- Anchovy paste
- Fresh lemon juice
- Worcestershire sauce
- Tabasco sauce
- Romaine or cos lettuce
- Canned anchovies
- Cauliflower
- Yellow mustard seed
- Jalapeno peppers
- Parsley
- Mushrooms
- Beef
- Red table wine
- Beef broth
- Sour cream
- Bacon
- Leeks
- Blue cheese or Roquefort cheese
- Butternut winter squash
- Yellow summer squash
- Pumpkin pie spice
- Tomato paste
- Paprika
- Oregano
- Cumin
- Boneless tuna
- Swiss chard

- Muenster cheese
- Eggplant
- Capers
- Cream cheese
- Mustard
- Original pepper sauce

One Week Meal Plan (Phase One)

Day One

Breakfast – Basque eggs with ham, tomatoes and bell peppers

Lunch – Asparagus drizzled with sun-dried tomato vinaigrette

Dinner – Chili beef stroganoff with a kick!

Day Two

Breakfast – Egg and mozzarella filled bell pepper rings

Lunch – Meatballs in the oven

Dinner – Creamy blue cheese and bacon soup

Day Three

Breakfast – Buttermilk waffles with cinnamon

Lunch – Classic bratwurst & sauerkraut

Dinner – Butternut squash soup

Day Four

Breakfast – Breakfast sausage sautéed with red & green bell peppers

Lunch – Basic yet delicious egg salad

Dinner – Cajun blackened tuna

Day Five

Breakfast – Cheesy onion omelette

Lunch – Buttered-up sprouts

Dinner - Chard and cheese casserole

Day Six

Breakfast – Cheesy eggs with a difference

Lunch – Caesar salad

Dinner – Caponata

Day Seven

Breakfast – Chocolate hazelnut smoothie

Lunch – Cauliflower salad

Dinner – Cauli cheese and mac

3

Phase One Recipes

Breakfast Recipes for Phase One

Eggs with Ham, Spicy Peppers & Tomatoes

Serves 2

Protein 19.6g, fat 30.2g, fiber 1.1g, calories 379, net carbs 6.9g

Ingredients

- Olive oil, 3 tablespoons
- Onion (medium), x 1
- Bell peppers, 8oz
- Tomatoes, x 2
- Basil, 5.5 tablespoons
- Cayenne pepper, 0.25 teaspoon

- Eggs x 12
- Unsalted butter, 6 tablespoons
- Cooked ham, 6oz
- Garlic, 3 teaspoons

Method

- Heat up the oil using a medium to high heat
- Cook the onions until soft for around five minutes
- Add the garlic to the mixture and continue cooking for an extra minute
- To the pan, add the cayenne pepper, the tomatoes and the peppers
- Put the lid on the pan and stir occasionally, for another 10 minutes
- Take the lid off the pan and simmer for around 10 minutes
- Add salt and pepper
- Beat the eggs in another bowl, to combine well
- Melt the butter over a low heat
- Place the eggs and basil into the pan and cook for ten minutes, stirring every so often
- Add the mixture with the peppers, as well as the ham and stir until mixed together
- Serve

Egg & Mozzarella Filled Bell Pepper Rings

Protein 18.7g, fat 19.9g, fiber 1g, calories 280, net carbs 5.1g
Serves 1 or 2

Ingredients

- Sweet red peppers (medium), x 2
- Eggs, x 2
- Canola vegetable oil, 1 teaspoon
- Mozzarella cheese (shredded), 0.25 cup

Method

- Cut the bell pepper into rings, removing the seeds as you go
- Heat the oil up over a medium heat
- Cook the rings
- Once cooked, crack an egg into each of the rings and cook it until it is exactly how you like it
- Once cooked, sprinkle the cheese on top and add a cover over the pan
- Cook for around one minute, until the cheese is melted
- Season and serve!

Buttermilk Waffles With Cinnamon

Protein 6.9g, fat 13g, fiber 1.4g, calories 166, net carbs 5.4g
Serves 2

Ingredients

- Whole grain soy flour, 1 cup
- Sweetener, 2 tablespoons

- Cinnamon, 2 teaspoons
- Baking powder, 3 teaspoons
- Baking soda, 0.5 teaspoons
- Buttermilk, 0.75 cup
- Unsalted butter, 6 tablespoons
- Eggs, x3
- Sugar free vanilla syrup, 1.5oz
- Tap water, 0.5 cup

Method

- Heat up the waffle pan
- In a bowl, mix together the soy flour, sweetener, spices, baking powder and soda
- Once combined, slowly add in the buttermilk and stir again
- Now add the butter, eggs and the syrup and blend until smooth
- A little at a time, add the cold water and continue stirring until you have a batter mixture
- Add the batter to the waffle pan
- Once the waffles are golden, they are cooked

Breakfast Sausage Sautéed with Red & Green Bell Peppers

Protein 25.7g, fat 33.4g, fiber 1.5g, calories 408, net carbs 3g
Serves 1

Ingredients

- Canola oil, 1 teaspoon
- Cooked turkey breakfast sausage, x 4
- Red sweet pepper
- Green sweet pepper
- Monterey Jack cheese, 1oz

Method

- Over a medium to high heat, add the oil to a skillet
- Add the sausage to the pan and brown for around 3 minutes
- Add the red and green peppers
- Cook for a further 5 minutes
- Sprinkle on the cheese to melt
- Serve

Cheesy Onion Omelette

Protein 26.7g, fiber 0.9g, fat 41.8g, calories 509, net carbs 6.8g
Serves 1

Ingredients

- Onions (chopped), 1/3 cup
- Extra virgin olive oil, 1 tablespoon
- Shredded cheddar cheese, 0.5 cup
- Eggs, x 2

Method

1. Heat the oil in the pan and cook the onions until translucent
2. Remove the onions from the pan
3. In a bowl, beat the eggs
4. Add the eggs to the pan and cook how you like, before flipping to cook the opposite side
5. Sprinkle the cheese to the omelette and allow to melt, cooking for another minute
6. Fold the omelette over in the pan
7. Cook for a further minute
8. Season with salt and pepper and serve

Cheesy Eggs With a Difference

Protein 17.1g, fiber 0g, fat 27.3g, calories 324, net carbs 2g
Serves 1

Ingredients

- Unsalted butter, 1 teaspoon
- Eggs, x 2
- Heavy cream, 2 tablespoons
- Parmesan cheese (grated), 2 tablespoons

Method

- Preheat the oven to 190°C
- Melt the butter in a dish which is suitable for the oven
- Mix together the eggs and cream in a separate bowl

- Add the cheese, ground black pepper and salt, mix together
- Pour the mixture into the oven-safe dish
- Bake for 10 minutes, until cooked and the cheese is bubbling
- Serve whilst still warm!

Chocolate Hazelnut Smoothie

Protein 23.2g, fiber 0g, fat 22.2g, calories 297, net carbs 3.2g
Serves 2

Ingredients

- Chocolate whey protein, 2 scoops
- Heavy cream, 1 tablespoon
- Sugar free hazelnut syrup, 12 teaspoons

Method

- Into a blend, place the protein powder, the cream and the syrup, as well as half a cup of ice
- Blend until totally combined
- Pour into glasses and serve

Lunch Recipes for Phase One

Asparagus Drizzled With Sun-Dried Tomato Vinaigrette

Protein 2.3g, fiber 2.2g, fat 7.1g, calories 87, net carbs 3.2g
Serves 2

Ingredients

- Asparagus spears, x 30
- Sun-dried tomatoes, 1.5oz
- Balsamic vinegar, 1 tablespoon
- Red wine vinegar, 1 tablespoon
- Garlic, 0.25 teaspoon
- Extra virgin olive oil, 3 tablespoons

Method

- Steam the asparagus for around 4 minutes, until tender
- Blend the remaining ingredients together until smooth
- Season the mixture with salt and vinegar
- Arrange the asparagus on a plate
- Drizzle the vinaigrette over the asparagus

Meatballs in the Oven

Protein 38.6g, fat 26.7g, fiber 0.2g, calories 409, net carbs 1.8g

Serves 2

Ingredients

- Extra virgin olive oil, 1 tablespoon
- Onion, spring onion works well
- Garlic, 1.5 teaspoons
- Ground veal, 0.5lb
- Ground beef, 0.5lb
- Ground pork, 0.5lb
- Grated parmesan cheese, 0.5 cup
- Eggs, x2
- Salt, 0.5 teaspoon
- Black pepper, 0.25 teaspoon

Method

- Pre-heat the oven to 190°C
- Cook the onion over a low heat until it is softened
- Once soft, add in the garlic and continue to cook for another minute
- Take a separate bowl and mix the meats together
- In another bowl, take the rest of the ingredients and combine them together
- Roll the meat mixture into small bowls, flattening down to make burgers/balls
- Place in the oven for 25-30 minutes

Classic Bratwurst & Sauerkraut

Protein 12.3g, fat 24.9g, fiber 1.9g, calories 297, net carbs 3.6g

Serves 1

Ingredients

- Bratwurst, x 1
- Canned sauerkraut, 0.5 cup

Method

- Preheat the grill using a medium heat
- Grill the bratwurst on all sides, until browned evenly
- Warm up the sauerkraut – a microwave oven works well for this
- Arrange the sauerkraut over the top of the Bratwurst and enjoy

Basic Yet Delicious Egg Salad

Protein 12.6g, fat 32.6g, fiber 0.5g, calories 363, net carbs 2.4g

Serves 2

Ingredients

- Eggs, x 8 – boiled to your liking
- Full fat mayonnaise, 0.5 cup
- Dijon mustard, 3 tablespoons
- Salt, 0.5 teaspoon
- Black pepper, 0.25 teaspoon
- Celery stalks, x 2

Method

- Take the eggs and boil them to the point that you like them and then chop up roughly
- Mix the eggs with the mayonnaise, mustard, salt and pepper
- Chop up the celery into rough, small pieces
- Add the celery to the egg mixture
- Arrange the mixture over a bed of lettuce and enjoy!

Buttered-up Sprouts

Protein 1.5g, fiber 1.7g, fat 5.9g, calories 70, net carbs 2.3g
Serves 4

Ingredients

- Brussels Sprouts, 2 cups
- Unsalted butter, 2 tablespoons

Method

- Cut the sprouts into halves and cook for around 7-8 minutes
- Once cooked, drain off the water and set aside to cool slightly
- Over a medium heat, melt the butter
- Once melted, add the sprouts to the buttered pan and toss well, to coat all sides

- Season to your liking
- Serve whilst warm

Caesar Salad

Protein 8.2g, fat 18.8g, fiber 3.4g, calories 224, net carbs 3.5g
Serves 4

Ingredients

- Real mayonnaise, 2 tablespoons
- Anchovy paste, 1 tablespoon
- Fresh lemon juice, 0.5 fluid oz
- Extra virgin olive oil, 1 tablespoon
- Worcestershire sauce, 0.5 tablespoon
- Garlic, 1 teaspoon
- Dijon mustard, 1 teaspoon
- Salt, 0.25 teaspoon
- Black pepper, 0.25 teaspoon
- Tabasco sauce, 1/8 teaspoon
- Grated parmesan cheese, 7 tablespoons
- Romaine or cos lettuce, 1 head
- Canned anchovies, x 8

Method

- Make the dressing first – take a small bowl and mix together the mayonnaise, anchovy paste, lemon juice, oil, Worcestershire sauce, garlic,

mustard, salt, pepper and the Tabasco. Mix together well
- Add in 3 tablespoons of cheese
- Toss in the lettuce and coat well
- Divide the mixture into plates
- Top with cheese
- Add 2 anchovies per plate

Cauliflower Salad

Protein 1.1g, fiber 1.2g, fat 5.7g, calories 66, net carbs 2.1g
Serves 8

Ingredients

- Cauliflower, 4 cups
- Real mayonnaise, 0.25 cups
- Fresh lemon juice, 2 tablespoons
- Yellow mustard seed, 0.5 teaspoons
- Chopped scallions or spring onions, 3 tablespoons
- Jalapeno pepper, x 1
- Salt, 0.5 teaspoon
- Black pepper, 1/8 teaspoon
- Parsley, 1 tablespoon

Method

- Cook the cauliflower in a large pot of salted water for 4-5 minutes
- Drain and rinse the cauliflower and pat dry

- Combine together the mayonnaise, lemon juice and the mustard
- Add the cauliflower, scallions, jalapeno, salt and black pepper together
- Mix the cauliflower into the sauce until totally coated
- Place in the refrigerator for around half an hour
- Serve with a sprinkling of parsley

Dinner Recipes for Phase One

Chili Beef Stroganoff With a Kick!

Protein 32g, fiber 0.4g, fat 24.3g, calories 379, net carbs 3.5g
Serves 8

Ingredients

- Brussel sprouts, x 10
- Brown mushrooms, 6oz
- Olive oil, 2 tablespoons
- Thyme, 2 teaspoons
- Paprika, 1 teaspoon
- Cinnamon, 1/8 teaspoon
- Garlic, 2 cloves
- Ground beef, 14oz
- Chili powder, 1 tablespoon
- Salt, 1 teaspoon
- Black pepper, 0.5 teaspoon
- Tomato paste, 2 tablespoons
- Sour cream, 0.25 cup

Method

- Bring a pan of water to the boil
- Halve the spouts and add them to the boiling water
- Add the oil to a skillet pan and allow to warm up
- Chop up the mushrooms
- Add the mushrooms to the pan and cook for 5 minutes
- To the pan, add the thyme, paprika, cinnamon and garlic and cook for half a minute more – keep stirring
- Remove the Brussel sprouts from the heat and drain
- Place the sprouts into serving plates
- Heat up the ground beef, seasoning with the chili powder, salt and pepper until brown
- Add the tomato paste to the beef pan and cook for a further 3 minutes
- Add the sour cream and stir in until it bubbles
- Serve the mixture over the sprouts

Creamy Blue Cheese and Bacon Soup

Protein 10.2g, fat 23.2g, fiber 1.3g, calories 274, net carbs 5.9g
Serves 6

Ingredients

- Bacon slices, x 6

- Unsalted butter, 3 tablespoons
- Leeks, x 2
- Mushrooms, 2 cups
- Cauliflower, 1.5 cups
- Canned chicken broth, 2 x 14.5oz cans
- Tap water, 0.5 cup
- Blue cheese, 2.5 oz (you can use Roquefort cheese if you prefer)

Method

- Over a medium to high heat, cook the bacon until crispy
- Pat dry with a paper towel to drain off the excess oil
- Over a medium heat and in a large pot, melt the butter
- Once melted, add the leeks, mushrooms and the cauliflower
- Cover and cook for 5 minutes, stirring every so often
- Add the chicken broth and the water
- Bring the pan to the boil
- Lower the heat and allow to simmer for a further 10 minutes
- Puree the soup in a blender or a food processor
- Add the soup back to the pot
- Add the blue cheese (or Roquefort) and puree again
- Heat over a low temperature once more
- Crumble the bacon over the top before serving

Butternut Squash Soup

Protein 3.3g, fat 12.6g, fiber 2.9g, calories 175, net carbs 12.5g
Serves 6

Ingredients

- Butternut winter squash, 1.25lbs
- Extra virgin olive oil, 2 tablespoons
- Yellow summer squash, 2 cups
- Onions (sliced), 0.25 cups
- Salt, 0.75 teaspoon
- Black pepper, 0.5 teaspoon
- Pumpkin pie spice, 1.5 tablespoons
- Tomato paste, 1 tablespoon
- Chicken broth, 2 x 14.5oz cans
- Heavy cream, 0.5 cup

Method

- Preheat the oven to 230°C
- Take the butternut squash and peel and cube it
- Toss the squash with 1 tablespoon of oil and half of the salt and pepper
- Take a baking sheet and roast the butter nut squash until it is softened slightly, around 15 minutes
- Toss the yellow squash and onions with the rest of the oil, the salt and pepper
- Add this to the baking tray and cook for 20 more minutes
- Take a large pot and simmer the pumpkin pie spice

and tomato paste, stirring all the time, for around 1 minute
- Add the vegetables and the broth to the large pot and bring to the boil
- Reduce the heat down to low and simmer for a further 20 minutes
- Remove from the heat
- Stir in the cream
- Puree the soup in a blender
- Season with salt and pepper
- Garnish with sour cream and serve

Cajun Blackened Tuna

Protein 26.8g, fat 8.6g, fiber 0.5g, calories 195, net carbs 0.7g
Serves 4

Ingredients

- Paprika, 0.5 tablespoon
- Oregano, 0.5 teaspoon
- Garlic powder, 0.5 teaspoon
- Onion powder, 0.5 teaspoon
- Salt, 0.5 teaspoon
- Black pepper, 0.25 teaspoon
- Cayenne pepper, 1/8 teaspoon
- Unsalted butter, 1 tablespoon
- Boneless tuna, 16oz

Method

- Preheat the oven to 200°C
- In a large bowl, mix together the paprika, oregano, garlic powder, onion powder, salt, cumin, pepper and cayenne pepper
- Transfer to a plate
- Rub the butter over the tuna steaks
- Press the steaks into the spice mixture and rub
- Heat a large skillet pan over a high heat, for around 2 minutes
- Cook the steaks one minute on each side
- Remove the skillet from the heat and transfer it to the oven
- Roast the tuna steaks until medium rare
- Cut the steaks in half and serve

Chard & Cheese Casserole

Protein 10.6g, fat 15.3g, fiber 1.6g, calories 195, net carbs 3.6g
Serves 6

Ingredients

- Extra virgin olive oil, 2 tablespoons
- Swiss chard, 0.75lb
- Sweet red peppers, x 1
- Onion, x 1
- Salt, 0.5 teaspoon

- Black pepper, 0.75 teaspoon
- Shredded Muenster cheese, 1.5 cups
- Parmesan cheese, 0.5 cups (grated)

Method

- Preheat the oven to 180°C
- Grease a baking dish, measuring around 13"
- In a large Dutch oven or a heavy pot, heat 1 tablespoon of oil
- Add the chard and cut for around 3-4 minutes
- Drin the chard and drain the excess liquid by pressing with the back of a spoon
- Heat the rest of the oil in a skillet pan over a medium heat
- Sauté the bell pepper and onion for around 8 minutes
- Mix in the chard and coat well with the mixture
- Season with salt and pepper
- Mix in the Muenster cheese
- Spoon the mixture into the dish you greased
- Sprinkle the parmesan cheese evenly over the top
- Cover the dish with aluminium foil
- Bake in the oven for around half an hour
- Take the foil off the dish and cook for a further 10 minutes

Caponata

Protein 0.9g, fat 9.5g, fiber 2.3g, calories 101, net carbs 2.7g

Serves 6

Ingredients

- Extra virgin olive oil, 0.25 cups
- Eggplant, 12oz
- Garlic, 0.5 teaspoon
- Sweet red peppers, 1 or 2 large
- Parsley, 2 tablespoons
- Water, 0.25 cup
- Salt, 1 teaspoon
- Red onion, 0.5
- Drained capers, 2 tablespoon
- Fresh lemon juice, 2 tablespoons

Method

- Heat the olive oil over a large saucepan
- Add the eggplant, bell pepper, onion, garlic and the water
- Bring to the boil and cover
- Simmer until the eggplant is tender and the water has mostly disappeared, stirring occasionally
- Mix in the salt, capers, parsley and lemon juice
- Cool the mixture down to room temperature and serve

Cauli Mac & Cheese

Protein 11.4g, fat 27.5g, fiber 3.6g, calories 320, net carbs 5.9g

Serves 6

Ingredients

- Cauliflower, x 1 large head
- Heavy cream, 1 cup
- Cream cheese, 2oz
- Mustard, 1.5 teaspoons
- Shredded cheddar cheese, 1.5 cups
- Garlic, 1 clove
- Salt, 1 teaspoon
- White pepper, 0.25 teaspoon
- Original pepper sauce, 0.25 teaspoon

Method

- Preheat the oven to 190°C
- Spray a baking dish with oil cooking spray (olive oil)
- Heat up a large pot of water and add 0.5 teaspoons of salt
- Remove the leaves and the stems from the cauliflower and cut into small pieces
- Place the cauliflower into the water and cook for around 5 minutes
- Drain well and pat dry with paper towels
- Bring the cream to a simmer in a pan
- Whisk in the cream cheese and powdered mustard to create a smooth texture

- Add the cheddar, minced garlic, salt, white pepper and pepper sauce
- Whisk until the cheese is melted
- Remove the pan from the heat and stir in the cauliflower
- Pour the mixture into the baking dish and cover with the rest of the cheese
- Bake for around 15 minutes, until bubbling and brown on top

4

Phase Two Shopping List & Meal Plan

Having come through phase one of the Atkins Diet, you should now be feeling slinky and slim, and the side effects you may have experienced in the first part of the diet should have disappeared, or at least improved dramatically.

Phase two is where you can begin to introduce foods with a slightly higher carb count than you could have in the first phase, but it's still very important to make sure you don't go over your allocated amount per day.

Shopping List for One Week of Phase Two

You may have accumulated a few of these ingredients from phase one, e.g. spices etc., so bear that in mind!

- Vanilla whey protein
- Almond meal flour
- Whole grain soy flour

- Baking powder
- Eggs
- Cottage cheese
- Greek yogurt
- Raspberries
- Almonds (blanched)
- Pure almond milk
- Ground beef
- Green chili peppers
- Garlic powder
- Chili powder
- Cumin
- Oregano leaves
- Salt
- Black pepper
- Bacon
- Cheddar cheese
- Cilantro
- Asparagus
- Heavy cream
- Parmesan cheese
- Garlic
- Corned beef brisket
- Turnips
- Onions
- Canola vegetable oil
- Coconut cream
- Vanilla whey protein
- Vanilla extract
- Extra virgin olive oil
- Baby spinach
- Artichokes

- Lemons
- Coriander seeds
- Unsalted butter
- Cucumber
- Blueberries
- Sweetener
- Rosemary
- Club soda
- Scallions or spring onions
- Broccoli
- White wine vinegar
- Celery
- Black olives
- Pumpkin
- Shallots
- Vegetable broth
- Sugar free syrup
- Sage
- Pork chops
- Monterey Jack cheese
- Green tomato Chile sauce (Salsa Verde)
- Jalapeno peppers
- Low carb tortillas
- Ground beef
- Red tomatoes
- Feta cheese
- Dill
- Sesame oil
- Chinese cabbage (bok choy)
- Crushed red pepper
- Peanuts
- Tamari soybean sauce

- Beef brisket
- Paprika
- Sugar free apricot preserve
- Artichokes
- Vegetable broth
- Fontina cheese
- Swiss cheese
- Parmesan cheese
- Avocados
- Ginger
- Zucchinis
- Endive
- Chives
- Goat's cheese
- Dijon mustard
- Atkins bread
- Romaine or cos lettuce
- Cheddar cheese
- Green sweet pepper
- Gorgonzola cheese
- Beef tenderloin
- Portobello mushrooms
- Canned tuna
- Real mayonnaise

One Week Meal Plan (Phase Two)

Day One

Breakfast – Almond pancakes

Lunch – Artichokes drizzled with lemon butter

Dinner – Apricot glazed brisket

Day Two

Breakfast – Almond raspberry smoothie

Lunch – Broccoli salad with olives

Dinner – Artichokes with three cheeses

Day Three

Breakfast – Beef huevos rancheros served with Canadian bacon

Lunch – Cucumber & blueberry freeze

Dinner – Avocado zucchini soup

Day Four

Breakfast – Baked eggs with asparagus

Lunch – Pumpkin spiced with sage and maple

Dinner – Bacon & goat's cheese salad

Day Five

Breakfast – Corned beef hash

Lunch – Spicy quesadillas

Dinner – Beef sauté

Day Six

Breakfast – Coconut vanilla shake

Lunch – Feta & tomato beef burger

Dinner – Beef fillet with bacon & gorgonzola butter

Day Seven

Breakfast – Eggs and spinach

Lunch – Chinese cabbage & onions

Dinner – Canned tuna & artichoke salad

5

Phase Two Recipes

Breakfast Recipes For Phase Two

Almond Pancakes

Protein 20g, fat 9.9g, fiber 1.6g, calories 191, net carbs 4.4g
Serves 4

Ingredients

- Vanilla whey protein, 2oz
- Almond meal flour, 0.25 cup
- Whole grain soy flour, 3 tablespoons
- Baking powder, 1 teaspoon
- Eggs, x 3
- Cottage cheese, 1/3 cup

Method

- You will need two bowls – in the first one, combine the whey powder, the almond meal, the soy flour and also the baking powder
- In the other bowl, add the cottage cheese and eggs, mixing together until totally combined
- Heat up the oil over a medium heat
- Using around a quarter of a cup of mixture per pancake, pour into the pan
- Once the pancake is ready to turn over, the mixture will bubble
- The pancakes are cooked when golden brown and spongey

Almond Raspberry Smoothie

Protein 18.1g, fat 17.8g, fiber 7.1g, calories 291, net carbs 10.8g
Serves 1

Ingredients

- Greek yogurt, 1 x 4oz container
- Raspberries, 0.5 cup
- Almonds (blanched and slivered), x 20
- Pure almond milk, 0.5 cup

Method

- Insert everything into a blender and puree/blend together until smooth

- Pour into a glass and enjoy!

Beef Huevos Rancheros Served With Canadian Bacon

Protein 23.1g, fat 15g, fiber 0.6g, calories 244, net carbs 2.5g
Serves 4

Ingredients

- Ground beef, 6 oz
- Green chili peppers, 0.5 cup
- Garlic powder, 0.25 teaspoon
- Chili powder, 1 teaspoon
- Cumin, 0.25 teaspoon
- Oregano, 0.25 teaspoon
- Salt, 0.25 teaspoon
- Black pepper, 0.25 teaspoon
- Canadian bacon, 4 slices
- Eggs, x 4
- Cheddar cheese (shredded), 0.5 cup
- Cilantro, x 4 leaves

Method

- Warm a pan over a medium heat and add the beef, cooking until brown
- Once browned, add in the chilies, the chili powder, the garlic, cumin, oregano, the salt and the pepper, combining well

- Cook for 10 minutes
- Once cooked, lie the bacon over the top of the beef and leave for around 5 minutes
- Remove the pan and set to one side
- Warm up the oil in another pan and add the eggs, cooking to your liking – scrambling is best here
- Place a slice of bacon on a plate, pile it with some beef and then the eggs on top
- Sprinkle cheese and cilantro over the top and enjoy

Baked Eggs and Asparagus

Protein 20.8g, fat 40.4g, fiber 4g, calories 471, net carbs 5.6g
Serves 1

Ingredients

- Asparagus, x 8 spears
- Heavy cream, 0.25 cup
- Eggs, x 2
- Almond meal flour, 2 tablespoons
- Parmesan cheese, 1 tablespoon
- Garlic, 1/8 teaspoon
- Black pepper, 1/8 teaspoon

Method

- Preheat the oven to 200°C
- Oil an oven-safe casserole dish to grease and set to one side

- Boil the asparagus for around 2 minutes, until tender but crisp
- Drain and pat dry
- Place the asparagus in the baking dish
- Pour the cream over the dish and then crack two of the eggs on top also
- In a separate dish, blend together the almond meal, parmesan cheese, black pepper and the garlic
- Sprinkle this mixture over the eggs
- Place in the oven and cook for around 5-10 minutes, to your liking

Corned Beef Hash

Protein 22g, fat 43.2g, fiber 1.9g, calories 506, net carbs 5.3g
Serves 4

Ingredients

- Corned beef brisket, 16oz
- Turnips, 2 cups
- Onions (chopped) 0.5 cup
- Heavy cream, 0.5 cup
- Canola vegetable oil, 3 tablespoons

Method

- Cut the turnips into cubes
- Cut the corned beef into cubes

- Toss the turnip and the corned beef together in a bowl with the onion and heavy cream
- Over a medium to low heat, heat the oil up in a non-stick skillet pan
- Add the mixture and cook for around 10 minutes, until a crust appears
- Turn over and cook on the other side for another 10 minutes
- Serve with a poached egg if you want to, but remember to add in the extra carbs for your allowance

Coconut Vanilla Shake

Protein 21.8g, fat 23.9g, fiber 0.6g, calories 310, net carbs 4g
Serves 4

Ingredients

- Coconut cream, 1 x 14oz can
- Vanilla whey protein, 2 scoops
- Vanilla extract, 0.5 teaspoon

Method

- Place everything into a blender as well as 2 cups of ice cubes and pulse until smooth
- Pour into a glass and serve

Eggs and Spinach

Protein 13.7g, fat 13.9g, fiber 1.3g, calories 194, net carbs 2.9g

Serves 1

Ingredients

- Extra virgin olive oil, 1 tablespoon
- Baby spinach, 1 x 1/16 cups
- Eggs, x 2

Method

- Warm up the oil in a small skillet pan, using a medium heat
- Add the spinach and cook until it has wilted
- Add the eggs and scramble to your liking
- Serve with salt and black pepper

Lunch Recipes For Phase Two

Artichokes Drizzled With Lemon Butter

Protein 4.8g, fat 23.7g, fiber 10g, calories 287, net carbs 9.9g

Serves 4

Ingredients

- Artichokes, x 4
- Lemons x 4

- Coriander seeds, 2 tablespoons
- Salt, 2 tablespoons
- Unsalted butter, 0.5 cup

Method

- Trim the artichokes and cut into pieces
- Bring a pan of water to the boil and cook the artichokes until tender
- Into some water, squeeze three of the lemons, keeping one aside
- Add the discarded lemon halves, the coriander seeds and the 2 tablespoons of salt
- Add the artichokes to the mixture and place a lid over the top to cover
- Return to the heat and cook for 15 minutes
- Remove the pan from the heat and drain off
- Melt the butter in a small pan and then add to a small bowl, mixing in the juice of the last lemon
- Season the mixture with salt and pepper and drizzle over the artichokes

Cucumber & Blueberry Freeze

Protein 0.7g, fat 0.3g, fiber 1.1g, calories 92, net carbs 5.3g
Serves 1

Ingredients

- Cucumber (chopped), 0.5 cup

- Lemon juice, 2 tablespoons
- Blueberries, 1 oz
- Sweetener, 0.5 teaspoon
- Rosemary, 1 teaspoon
- Ice cubes, x 4
- Club soda, 4oz

Method

- Cut the cucumber up into tiny pieces and blend to further cut it down
- Into the blender, add the lemon juice, the blueberries and the sweetener and combine
- Add the rosemary into the blender and pulse
- Strain the mixture to get rid of the pulp
- Take a serving glass and add in the ice cubes and club soda
- Pour the mixture into the glass and stir well

Broccoli Salad with Olives

Protein 2g, fat 19.2g, fiber 2.7g, calories 198, net carbs 3.4g
Serves 4

Ingredients

- Scallions or spring onions, x 2
- Broccoli flower clusters, 3 cups
- Garlic, 0.5 teaspoon
- White wine vinegar, 2 tablespoons

- Capers (drained), 1 tablespoon
- Salt, 0.5 teaspoon
- Extra virgin olive oil, 1/3 cup
- Celery stalk, x 3
- Black olives x 6
- Black pepper, 0.25 teaspoon

Method

- Steam the broccoli until crisp but tender
- Drain the broccoli and rinse it out under cold water
- Take a blender or a food processor and combine the garlic, vinegar, capers, salt,\ and pepper
- Add the oil gradually and continue to blend until the mixture is smooth
- Pour the dressing into a large bowl
- Slice up the broccoli into thin pieces and add to the dressing
- Add the celery, scallions/spring onions and the olives
- Toss to ensure everything is coated
- Serve

Pumpkin Spiced With Sage & Maple

Protein 0.6g, fat 1.2g, fiber 0.4g, calories 26, net carbs 3.5g
Serves 8

Ingredients

- Pumpkin, 1lb
- Shallots, chopped, 0.25 cup
- Unsalted butter, 1 tablespoon
- Vegetable broth, 0.25 cup
- Sugar free syrup, 1/16 cup
- Ground sage, 0.25 teaspoon

Method

- Melt the butter over a medium to high heat
- Take the pumpkin and cut roughly into chunks of around ¾ of an inch
- Add the shallots to the pan
- Add the pumpkin to the pan and cook them together for around 5 minutes, until the pumpkin has turned just brown and the shallots are clear
- Lower the heat and pour in the vegetable broth, covering the pan
- Simmer the contents for 10 minutes more
- Add the maple syrup and stir to combine
- Add the sage and stir to combine

Spicy Quesadillas

Protein 43.4g, fat 40.3g, fiber 1g, calories 569, net carbs 5.1g
Serves 4

Ingredients

- Olive oil, 2 tablespoons

- Onions (chopped), 2 tablespoons
- Pork chops, 16oz
- Monterey Jack cheese, 1oz
- Salsa verde, 0.25 cup
- Jalapeno pepper, x 1
- Coriander, 0.25 cup
- Black pepper, 1 teaspoon
- Salt 0.25 teaspoon
- Low carb tortilla x 1

Method

- Preheat the oven to 230°C
- In a large pan, heat up 1 tablespoon of the oil
- Cook the onion for 5 minutes, until soft and translucent
- Remove the onion from the pan and transfer it to a bowl
- Add the pork to the bowl, as well as the cheese, salsa, jalapeno, cilantro, pepper and the salt, combining everything together well
- Brush one side of the tortilla with the oil lightly
- On the opposed side of the tortilla, add the mixture and distribute it evenly across the surface
- Fold the tortilla in half carefully
- Place in the oven for 5 minutes, until the cheese has melted and the tortilla has gone a little crunchy

Feta & Tomato Beef Burger

Protein 24.3g, fat 13.4g, fiber 0.5g, calories 231, net carbs 1.3g
Serves 4

Ingredients

- Ground beef, 1lb
- Spring onion, x 1
- Baby spinach, 0.5 cup
- Sliced or chopped tomatoes, 0.25 cup
- Crumbled feta cheese, 0.25 cup
- Dill (fresh), 1.5 teaspoons
- Salt, 0.5 teaspoon
- Black pepper, 0.5 teaspoon

Method

- Combine the beef, spring onion, tomato, feta, salt, pepper and dill in a bowl
- Split the meat mixture up into four and create a burger shape
- Heat up a pan over a medium heat
- Cook the burgers for 5-6 minutes on one side
- Turn the burgers and cook on the other side for another 5-6 minutes

Chinese Cabbage & Onions

Protein 3.5g, fat 8.3g, fiber 1.4g, calories 100, net carbs 3.3g
Serves 4

Ingredients

- Spring onions/scallions, x 4
- Water, 1 fluid oz
- Sweetener, 1 teaspoon
- Canola vegetable oil, 1 tablespoon
- Sesame oil, 1 teaspoon
- Chinese cabbage, 8 large pieces (Bok Choy works well for this recipe)
- Garlic, 1.5 teaspoons
- Red pepper, crushed, 1/8 teaspoons
- Peanuts in the shell, 1 cup
- Tamari soybean sauce, 2 tablespoons

Method

- Mix together the tamari soybean sauce, the water and sweetener
- Heat up the oils in a large pan
- Add the Chinese cabbage, garlic, pepper and the soy sauce and cook for around 3 minutes
- Add in the peanuts and stir to distribute well
- Enjoy whilst still warm

Dinner Recipes For Phase Two

Apricot Glazed Brisket

Protein 47.1g, fat 16.8g, fiber 0.3g, calories 358, net carbs 1.3g
Serves 8

Ingredients

- Beef brisket, 4lb
- Salt, 2 teaspoons
- Paprika, 2 teaspoons
- Black pepper, 1 teaspoon
- Sugar free apricot preserve, 3 tablespoons

Method

- Preheat the oven to 240°C
- Season the brisket with the pepper, paprika and salt
- Cook the brisket in the oven for around 15 minutes, with the onions and carrots
- Turn the brisket to the fat side upwards and add half a cup of water
- Cover the container
- Reduce the temperature of the oven down to 190°C
- Cook the meat for 3 to 4 hours, until tender
- Heat the broiler
- Spread the apricot preserve over the meat
- Place the meat in the broiler for 5 minutes, until the preserve changes color to brown
- Remove the carrots and onions from the other tray
- Allow to rest before serving with the remaining juices

Artichokes With Three Cheeses

Protein 11.5g, fat 21.5g, fiber 1.1g, calories 250, net carbs 2.8g
Serves 4

Ingredients

- Artichokes, 1 x 9oz packet
- Vegetable broth, 0.5 cup
- Extra virgin olive oil, 3 tablespoons
- Garlic, 3 teaspoons
- Parsley, 2 tablespoons
- Fresh lemon juice, 1 teaspoon
- Fontina cheese (shredded) 0.5 cup
- Basil, x 6 leaves
- Swiss cheese (shredded), 0.5 cup
- Parmesan cheese (grated) 0.5 cup

Method

- Preheat the oven to 200°C
- Take an 11 x 7" baking dish and arrange the artichokes on it
- Drizzle with olive oil and lemon juice
- Sprinkle with the basil and the parsley
- Cover with dish with the cheeses
- Cover the dish with aluminium foil
- Place in the oven and bake until artichokes are tender and the cheeses have melted (around 15 minutes should be enough)
- Uncover the dish and continue to bake for another 25 minutes
- Remove from oven and allow to cool before serving

Avocado Zucchini Soup

Protein 2.4g, fat 12.6g, fiber 4g, calories 156, net carbs 7.4g
Serves 4

Ingredients

- Avocado, skinned and de-seeded
- Extra virgin olive oil, 2 tablespoons
- Scallions or spring onions, x 4
- Ginger, 1 teaspoon
- Garlic, 1 x clove
- Zucchinis, x 2
- Vegetable brother, 29oz
- Tap water, 1 cup
- Salt, 0.5 teaspoon
- Black pepper, 0.5 teaspoon
- Lemon juice, 1 tablespoon
- Sweet red peppers (chopped), 1/16 cup

Method

- Over a medium heat, warm up the oil in a large pan
- Add 2/3 of the onions and cook for around 3 minutes
- Add in the ginger and stir for a further 1 minute
- Add the broth, water, zucchini, salt and the pepper and combine, cooking for 10 minutes
- Allow to cool for a few minutes

- Add in the avocado
- Puree the soup in a blender or food processor
- Return the soup to the heat and stir in the lemon juice
- Serve with red pepper and the rest of the onions

Bacon & Goat's Cheese Salad

Protein 13.8g, fat 27.8g, fiber 1.8g, calories 320, net carbs 2.7g
Serves 6

Ingredients

- Endive (chopped), 2 cups
- Chives (chopped), 3 tablespoons
- Goat's cheese, 8oz
- Extra virgin olive oil, 2 tablespoons
- Egg, x 1
- Red wine vinegar, 1.5 tablespoons
- Dijon mustard, 1 tablespoon
- Atkins bread, 1.5 pieces
- Black pepper, 0.75 teaspoon
- Cos or romaine lettuce (shredded), 4 cups
- Bacon, x 6 medium slices

Method

- Over a medium heat, cook the bacon in a skillet pan until crisp

- Blot with paper towel to remove the excess fat after cooking
- In a large mixing bowl, mix together the romaine, endive and the chives
- Make bread crumbs with the bread, using a food processor or a blender
- Place the crumbs on a plate
- Flatten the goat's cheese
- Dip each slice of cheese into the egg and allow the excess to drip away
- Now press the cheese into the crumbs and coat completely
- Over a medium heat, place the goat's cheese into a medium skillet pan and cook for 2 minutes on each side, until brown
- Keep the bacon drippings and combine with the olive oil, vinegar, mustard and pepper, placing it all in the skillet pan
- Arrange the cheese on a plate and add the lettuce mixture and the dressing
- Serve

Beef Sauté

Protein 43.5g, fat 47.1g, fiber 2g, calories 628, net carbs 6g
Serves 1

Ingredients

- Onions (chopped), 0.25 cup

- Extra virgin olive oil, 1 tablespoon
- Green sweet pepper (chopped), 0.5 cup
- Cheddar cheese (shredded), 0.5 cup
- Ground beef, 5oz

Method

- Brown the beef with a small amount of oil until brown, this should take no more than two minutes
- Combine the bell pepper and onions into the meat mixture and mix together well
- Cook for a little more time, until the meat is cooked and the vegetables are soft
- Season to your liking
- Serve immediately, pouring off any excess fat beforehand
- Sprinkle the cheese on top and allow it to melt

Beef Fillet With Bacon & Gorgonzola Butter

Protein 40.1g, fat 59.7g, fiber 1.9g, calories 747, net carbs 10.8g
Serves 2

Ingredients

- Scallions or spring onions, x 1
- Unsalted butter, 2 tablespoons
- Gorgonzola cheese, 1oz
- Beef tenderloin, 12oz

- Salt, 0.25 teaspoon
- Black pepper, 0.25 teaspoon
- Bacon, x 2 slices
- Extra virgin olive oil, 2 teaspoons
- Portobello mushroom caps, 8oz

Method

- Preheat the oven to 220°C
- Finely chop the green part of the scallion or spring onion and stir with the butter and cheese
- Take the beef fillets and season with salt and pepper
- Wrap a bacon slice around each fillet and hold it in place with a toothpick
- Heat the oil over a medium to high heat, using a non-stick skillet pan
- Add the meat to the pan and cook on both sides until browned, around 5 minutes each side
- Transfer the fillets to a baking sheet and place in the oven for 7-10 minutes
- Using the skillet pan you just cooked the beef in, add the mushrooms, the rest of the scallion and salt and pepper
- Reduce the heat down to low and stir, making sure the mushroom cook until tender, for around 4 minutes
- Spoon the mushroom mixture onto the fillets
- Serve with the Gorgonzola butter mixture

Canned Tuna & Artichoke Salad

Protein 32.7g, fat 33.7g, fiber 3.5g, calories 464, net carbs 4.1g
Serves 1

Ingredients

- Canned tuna, 4oz
- Artichoke hearts (marinated), x 6
- Real mayonnaise, 2 tablespoons
- Cos or romaine lettuce (shredded), 2 cups

Method

- Drain the tuna
- Mix together the tuna with the chopped up artichoke hearts and the mayonnaise
- Season with salt and pepper
- Serve the mixture over the lettuce leaves

6

Phase Three Shopping List & Meal Plan

By the time you have reached phase three, you are well on your way to your target weight and a healthier weight and lifestyle! Well done for getting this far and the end is in sight!

In terms of recipes, you can now start to introduce more in the way of carbs, but again, keep an eye on the scales to see how your body reacts to it.

Shopping List For One Week of Phase Three

Again, remember that a lot of the items on this shopping list will have been bought during the first phase or two of the diet.

- Plain yogurt (whole milk)
- Pineapple
- Almonds (blanched)
- Pure almond milk

- Pork & beef chorizo
- Ground beef
- Onions
- Cheddar cheese
- Eggs
- Sweet red peppers
- Creamy chocolate shake mixture
- Heavy cream
- Instant coffee powder
- Cayenne pepper
- Canola vegetable oil
- Scallions or spring onions
- Jalapeno peppers
- Low carb tortillas
- Tabasco sauce
- Salsa
- Chili powder
- Garlic powder
- Cumin
- Green chili peppers (canned)
- Light turkey meat
- Oregano leaves
- Bacon
- Turkey sausage
- High protein TVP (Textured Vegetable Protein)
- Celery
- Carrots
- Chicken broth
- Frozen spinach
- Ground turkey
- Thyme
- Sweet green pepper

- Nutmeg
- Cider vinegar
- Celery salt
- Chicken wings
- Blue cheese or Roquefort cheese
- Cucumber
- Original hummus
- Mushrooms
- Tamari soybean sauce
- Serrano pepper
- Tomatoes
- Silken tofu
- Chinese cabbage
- Green Cauliflower
- Kalamata olives
- Chicken breasts
- Feta cheese
- Fennel bulk
- Gruyere cheese
- Low carb baking mix
- Pears
- Vanilla extract
- Fresh ham (cooked)
- Brie cheese
- Sun-dried tomatoes
- Dried pine nuts
- Pork chops (bone in)
- Leaf tarragon
- Green peas
- Pesto sauce

Meal Plan For One Week of Phase Three

Day One

Breakfast – Tropical smoothie

Lunch – Chicken wings, Buffalo-style

Dinner – Red wine chicken

Day Two

Breakfast – Breakfast peppers, Mexican-style

Lunch – Cucumber with hummus

Dinner – Baked brie with sun-dried tomatoes & pine nuts

Day Three

Breakfast – Chocolate coffee frappe

Lunch – Vegetables, Asian-style

Dinner – Cajun pork chops

Day Four

. . .

Breakfast – Breakfast burrito

Lunch – Cauliflower Salad

Dinner – Asparagus tarragon cream soup

Day Five

Breakfast – Farmers breakfast Soup

Lunch – Greek salad with chicken

Dinner – Asparagus, mushrooms & peas

Day Six

Breakfast – Turkey wrapped breakfast tacos

Lunch – Baked fennel au grain

Dinner - Cauliflower with red pepper and black olives

Day Seven

Breakfast – Turkey breakfast meatloaf

Lunch – Baked pear fan

Dinner – Chicken pesto salad

7

Phase Three Recipes

Breakfast Recipes for Phase Three

Tropical Smoothie

Protein 10.8g, fat 18.6g, fiber 4.2g, calories 280, net carbs 17g
Serves 1

Ingredients

- Yogurt (plain), 0.5 cup
- Pineapple, 2.5 oz
- Almonds (whole), x 20
- Almond milk (the pure variety), 0.5 cup

Method

- Blend all ingredients together until smooth
- Pour into a glass and serve!

Breakfast Peppers, Mexican Style

Protein 21.3g, fat 20.1g, fiber 1.5g, calories 298, net carbs 5.3g
Serves 4

Ingredients

- Beef and pork chorizo, 4oz
- Ground beef, 4 oz
- Onions (chopped), 0.5 cup
- Cheddar cheese (shredded), 0.25 cup
- Eggs, x 3
- Red peppers (the sweet versions), x 2

Method

- Preheat the oven to 200°C
- Prepare a baking tray by lining it with aluminium foil
- Brown the chorizo
- Transfer the chorizo into a bowl and add in the beef, mixing together well
- To the bowl, add the eggs, onion and cheese, and combine everything together
- Prepare the peppers by cutting in half and removing the seeds

- Stuff each pepper half with some of the mixture – be generous!
- Place in the oven for half an hour

Chocolate Coffee Frappe

Protein 11.3g, fat 25.7g, fiber 7g, calories 302, net carbs 5.5g
Serves 1

Ingredients

- Creamy chocolate shake mixture, 11 fluid ozs
- Heavy cream, 3 tablespoons
- Instant coffee powder, 3 teaspoon

Method

- Add the creamy chocolate shake powder with two cups of ice, the cream and the instant coffee
- Place all in a blender and combine until the ice has been crushed
- Serve with extra cream if you want to

Breakfast Burrito

Protein 17.8g, fat 19.2g, fiber 5g, calories 281, net carbs 7.9g
Serves 2

Ingredients

- Salt, 0.5 teaspoon
- Cayenne pepper, 0.25 teaspoon
- Canola oil, 1 tablespoon
- Eggs x 4
- Sweet red peppers, 3 teaspoons
- Spring onions, 2 tablespoons
- Jalapeno pepper, x1
- Low carb tortillas, x2
- Tabasco sauce, 1/8 teaspoon
- Salsa, 2oz

Method

- Whisk together the eggs, cayenne and salt
- Over a medium heat, toast the tortillas for a minute, turning halfway through
- Cook the oil, red pepper, spring onion and jalapeno until soft
- Add the eggs and stir, cooking for around 2 minutes more
- Divide the mixture between the tortillas evenly

Farmers Breakfast Soup

Protein 26.8g, fat 14.4g, fiber 3.6g, calories 277, net carbs 5g
Serves 4

Ingredients

- Onions (chopped), 0.5 cup
- Bacon, x 2 medium slices
- Turkey sausage, 8oz
- Ground beef, 4oz
- High protein TVP, 2/3 cup
- Celery (chopped), 0.5 cup
- Carrots (chopped), 0.5 cup
- Chicken broth, 4 cups
- Black pepper, 0.25 teaspoon

Method

- Over a medium heat, cook the bacon until brown
- Add the sausage and beef, breaking up into smaller pieces and until brown
- Stir in the TVP and the other vegetables
- Cook for around 5 minutes, until the vegetables are soft
- Add the rest of the ingredients which are left and allow to simmer for around 20 minutes
- Keep removing the excess fat which appears on the top of the soup
- Season with salt and pepper
- Serve

Turkey Wrapped Breakfast Tacos

Protein 27.1g, fat 17.2g, fiber 0.7g, calories 285, net carbs 4g
Serves 6

Ingredients

- Onions (chopped), 0.5 cup
- Canola vegetable oil, 1 tablespoon
- Chili powder, 1 teaspoon
- Garlic powder, 0.25 teaspoon
- Cumin, 0.25 teaspoon
- Green chili peppers (canned), 2/3 cup
- Eggs, x 3
- Ground beef, 1lb
- Light turkey meat, 1 oz
- Oregano leaves, 0.25 teaspoon

Method

- Over a medium heat, cook the onion, beef and the spices together for around 20 minutes
- Stir the eggs into the mixture and allow to cook until they are firm
- Remove the pan from the heat and put the content into a serving dish
- Using the turkey, make the shape of a taco, and spoon inside the mixture, before folding up to secure
- Serve

Turkey Breakfast Meatloaf

Protein 36.6g, fat 25.6g, fiber 2.3g, calories 386, net carbs 2.8g

Serves 8

Ingredients

- Frozen spinach (chopped), 1 x 10oz packet
- Celery, 4 x stalks
- Sweet red peppers, x 1
- Turkey breakfast sausage, 24oz
- Ground turkey, 1.5 lbs
- Eggs, x 6
- Onion, x 1
- Ground thyme (dried), 0.5 teaspoon
- Green sweet pepper, x 1
- Nutmeg (ground), 1/8 teaspoon
- Cayenne pepper, 1/8 tablespoon

Method

- Preheat the oven to 170°C
- Chop the spinach roughly
- Dice up the celery, bell peppers and the onions
- Mix together the turkey sausage, the spinach, celery, onions and bell peppers
- Add the eggs, cayenne, thyme, nutmeg, garlic powder and season with salt and pepper
- Distribute the mixture evenly between two bread pans (about 4x9")
- Bake until cooked through and brown on top, around one hour

Phase Three Lunch Recipes

Chicken Wings, Buffalo-style

Protein 30.8g, fat 78.2g, fiber 0.2g, calories 848, net carbs 1.9g
Serves 6

Ingredients

- Cider vinegar, 1 cup
- Canola vegetable oil, 0.5 cup
- Black pepper, 0.5 teaspoon
- Garlic powder, 0.5 teaspoon
- Salt, 1 teaspoon
- Celery salt, 0.25 teaspoon
- Cayenne pepper, 1/8 teaspoon
- Chicken wings, 32oz
- Egg, x 1
- Full fat mayonnaise, 1 cup
- Sour cream, 0.5 cup
- Spring onions or 1 scallion
- Blue cheese, 1/3 cup
- Lemon juice, 0.5 fluid oz

Method

- Preheat the oven to 230°C
- Combine together the egg, vinegar, salt, oil, pepper, garlic powder, celery salt and cayenne into a small bowl

- Dip each piece of chicken into the bowl with the mixture in and arrange on a baking tray
- Place the tray in the oven and cook for around half an hour, remembering to turn the chicken over every so often
- In a separate bowl, add the mayonnaise, sour cream, cheese, scallion/spring onion, lemon juice and garlic and combine together well
- Arrange the cooked chicken on a plate, with the dipping sauce in a separate bowl

Cucumbers & Hummus

Protein 5.4g, fat 5.9g, fiber 4.1g, calories 115, net carbs 8.2g
Serves 1

Ingredients

- Cucumber (sliced), 1 cup
- Organic hummus (classic), 4 tablespoons

Method

- Slice the cucumber into pieces
- Dip into the hummus and enjoy

Vegetables, Asian-Style

Protein 6.7g, fat 2.1g, fiber 1.8g, calories 65, net carbs 4.6g
Serves 6

Ingredients

- Spring onions/scallions, 3 cups
- Mushrooms, 2 cups
- Tamari soybean sauce, 4 tablespoons
- Ginger, 3 teaspoons
- Garlic, 1 clove
- Serrano pepper, x1
- Red tomato (sliced), 1 cup
- Firm Tofu, 6oz
- Carrot
- Cilantro, 0.5oz
- Chinese cabbage (shredded), 2 cups
- Chicken broth, 6 cups

Method

- Bring to the boil the broth and tamari in a large pan
- Turn down the heat and add the Chinese cabbage, mushrooms, ginger, garlic and chili
- Simmer for around 5 minutes
- Add the tomatoes, onions, tofu and carrot, cook for around 1 minute more
- Stir in the cilantro and serve whilst still warm

Cauliflower Salad

Protein 2.9g, fat 7.7g, fiber 3.1g, calories 101, net carbs 3.8g
Serves 6

Ingredients

- Spring onions, x 3
- Mayonnaise, 4 tablespoons
- Lemon juice, 1 fluid oz
- Sugar substitute, 1 teaspoon
- Ground mustard, 0.5 teaspoon
- Cauliflower head x 1
- Jalapeno pepper x1
- Salt, 1/8 teaspoon
- Black pepper, 1/8 teaspoon

Method

- Cook the cauliflower in salted water
- Drain and pat dry
- Mix together the mayonnaise, lemon juice, sugar substitute and the mustard
- Add the cauliflower, pepper and onion
- Mix together until well coated
- Season with salt and pepper

Greek Salad With Chicken

Protein 27.2g, fat 29g, fiber 4.4g, calories 416, net carbs 9.7g
Serves 2

Ingredients

- Garlic, x 1 clove
- Red wine vinegar, 1.5 tablespoons
- Oregano, 1 teaspoon
- Cucumber, 0.5
- Shallots, 1oz
- Tomato, x 1
- Cos or Romaine lettuce, 0.5 head
- Kalamata olives, x 6
- Chicken breast, 12oz
- Feta cheese (crumbled), 0.25 cup
- Olive oil, 2 1/3 tablespoons
- Salt, 0.5 teaspoon
- Black pepper, 0.5 teaspoon

Method

- Chop up the garlic and put it in a small bowl
- Mix in with vinegar, oregano, half a tablespoon of water and quarter a tablespoon each of salt and pepper
- Add in two tablespoons of oil and mix well
- Cut the cucumber lengthwise
- Put half of the cucumber into a large bowl
- Cut the shallow into thin slices and add in with the cucumber
- Chop up the tomato into half an inch pieces and add in
- Chop the lettuce into 1" pieces and add to the bowl
- Cut the olives in half and add into the bowl, place the bowl to one side

- Season the chicken with 0.25 teaspoon each of salt and pepper
- Sauté the thicken over a medium to high heat for around 4 minutes on each side
- Remove from the heat and place the chicken on a plate
- Cut the chicken into slices and set aside
- Mix up the salad to ensure it is evenly coated
- Serve with the chicken and salad together
- Crumble the feta cheese over the top

Baked Fennel au Gratin

Protein 8.1g, fat 26.4g, fiber 2.7g, calories 293, net carbs 5g
Serves 6

Ingredients

- Fennel bulk, x 2 bulbs
- Salt, 0.5 teaspoon
- Black pepper, 0.25 teaspoon
- Heavy cream, 1 cup
- Gruyere cheese (shredded), 0.5 cup
- Parmesan cheese (grated), 2 tablespoons
- All purpose low-carb baking mix, 0.5 serving
- Unsalted butter, 0.25 cup

Method

- Preheat the oven to 200°C

- Prepare a shallow baking dish by greasing all sides
- Trim the fennel, leaving just the stalk, quarter the bulbs and remove the core. Cut into quarter slices
- Cook the fennel over a medium heat until tender, for around 10 minutes
- Drain and season with salt and pepper
- Transfer the fennel into a baking dish and press down to form an even layer
- Melt the butter over a medium heat
- Stir in 3 tablespoons of the baking mix and cook for 2 minutes
- Add the cream and bring to the boil
- Whisk constantly whilst cooking for a further 4 minutes
- Turn off the heat
- Stir in the gruyere until it has all melted
- Pour the mixture over the fennel and sprinkle the dish with the parmesan cheese
- Cover the dish with aluminium foil and bake for 15 minutes
- Take the covering off and bake for a further 15-20 minutes until golden brown and bubbling

Baked Pear Fan

Protein 0.4g, fat 3g, fiber 2.9g, calories 80, net carbs 11.5
Serves 4

Ingredients

- Pears, x 2
- Unsalted butter, 1 tablespoon
- Fresh lemon juice, 1 tablespoon
- Black pepper, 0.25 teaspoon
- Ginger, 0.25 teaspoon
- Cinnamon, 0.25 teaspoon
- Water, 1 fluid oz
- Vanilla extract, 0.25 teaspoon

Method

- Preheat the oven to 200°C
- Cut each pair into halves, starting 1/3" from the stem and cutting down to the rounded part to make the fans
- Melt the butter in a square baking dish over a medium heat
- Add the lemon juice, pepper, ginger, water and cinnamon, combining well
- Place the pears into the pan, with the rounded side pointing upwards
- Cover the pan with aluminium foil and bake until they are tender, for about 40 minutes
- Turn the pears after 20 minutes
- Transfer the pears onto serving plates and fan them out
- Stir the vanilla into the plan and cook over a medium heat for around one minute
- Spoon over the pears and serve

Dinner Recipes For Phase Three

Red Wine Chicken

Protein 48.3g, fat 16.8g, fiber 0.9g, calories 392, net carbs 3.5g
Serves 4

Ingredients

- Celery, x 1
- Olive oil, 2 tablespoons
- Carrot, 0.5
- Garlic, 1 teaspoon
- Parsley, 2 tablespoons
- Chicken broth, 0.5 cup
- Red wine, 4 fluid oz
- Cooked chicken thighs, 32oz
- Onion, x 1
- Bay leaf (crumbled), 0.5 teaspoon
- Fresh cooked ham, 2oz

Method

- Warm up the oil over a medium heat
- Cook the onion, carrot and celery until everything has softened
- Now add the ham and garlic, mixing together and cooking for a further 2 minutes
- Remove the mixture from the pan and place it in a bowl, to one side

- Cook the chicken thighs well on all sides, ensuring they are cooked and brown
- Add the wine, broth and the crumbled bay leaf to the pan
- Turn the heat down to medium/low
- Cook for half an hour – the liquid should reduce a little
- Return to the pan the mixture you placed in a separate bowl
- Combine everything together and cook for another 5 minutes

Baked Brie With Sun-Dried Tomatoes & Pine Nuts

Protein 8.1g, fat 11.6g, fiber 0.1g, calories 138, net carbs 0.5g
Serves 6

Ingredients

- Brie cheese, 8oz
- Chopped sun-dried tomatoes, 1 tablespoon
- Parsley, 1 tablespoon
- Dried pine nuts, 0.5 oz

Method

- Preheat the oven to 230°C
- Remove the rind from the cheese

- In a bowl combine the sun-dried tomatoes and the parsley
- Spread the mixture over the cheese evenly, in a thick layer
- Sprinkle the pine nuts over the top
- Place in the oven for 10 minutes, until the cheese has melted
- Serve whilst warm

Brisket With Mushrooms

Serves 10

Ingredients

- Dried Porcini mushrooms, 15 pieces
- Extra virgin olive oil, 1 tablespoon
- Beef brisket, 4lb
- Onion x 2
- Garlic, 1.5 teaspoons
- Beef broth, 1 can/14oz
- Crumbled Bay leaf, 1 teaspoon
- Salt, 0.5 teaspoon
- Black pepper, 0.25 teaspoon

Method

- Into a small bowl add the mushrooms and the water

- Microwave the mixture until boiling and then allow to cool
- Over a medium heat, warm up the oil
- Take the brisket and warm it on one side, turn over and add the onions
- Add the garlic when the onions are brown, cook for a further one minute
- Take the mushrooms from the liquid (keep the liquid to one side)
- Rinse the mushrooms and chop roughly
- Place the mushrooms to the brisket
- Strain the reserved liquid from the mushrooms and add to the brisket mixture
- Add the broth, Bay leaf, salt and pepper
- Cover the mixture and reduce the heat down to low
- Cook for just over two hours and then remove the brisket
- Turn the heat up and cook until the juices are thickened
- Cut the brisket into slices and serve with the mixture

Cajun Pork Chops

Protein 16.2g, fat 10.2g, fiber 0.9g, calories 165, net carbs 0.7g
Serves 4

Ingredients

- Paprika, 1 tablespoon
- Cumin, 0.5 teaspoon
- Ground sage, 0.5 teaspoon
- Black pepper, 0.5 teaspoon
- Garlic powder, 0.5 teaspoon
- Cayenne pepper, 0.5 teaspoon
- Pork chops, 24oz
- Unsalted butter, 0.5 tablespoon
- Canola oil, 0.5 tablespoon

Method

- Combine all the spices onto a plate
- Press the pork chops into the seasonings, on both sides
- On a high heat, melt the butter and oil
- Cook the chops in the skillet on a medium heat for just under 5 minutes on each side
- Serve

Asparagus Tarragon Cream Soup

Protein 3.9g, fat 10.5g, fiber 2.9g, calories 128, net carbs 4g
Serves 8

Ingredients

- Extra virgin olive oil, 1 tablespoon
- Chicken broth, 3 x 14.5 oz cans
- Asparagus, 2lbs

- Celery, 3 x stalks
- Salt, 0.25 teaspoon
- Black pepper, 0.25 teaspoon
- Onion, x 1
- Tarragon, 0.5 tablespoon (leaf)
- Heavy cream, 0.75 cup

Method

- Over a medium to high heat, warm up the oil
- Add the onion and cook for around 5 minutes
- Add the broth, asparagus, celery, salt, pepper and half of the tarragon
- Bring the pot to the boil
- Lower the heat and allow to simmer for around 20 minutes, until the asparagus is tender
- Blend the soup until smooth
- Return the soup to the pot
- Add the cream and the rest of the tarragon
- Heat the soup up
- Season with salt and pepper

Asparagus, Mushrooms & Peas

Protein 3g, fat 7.8g, fiber 2.6g, calories 103, net carbs 3.8g
Serves 6

Ingredients

- Unsalted butter, 3 tablespoons

- Scallions or spring onions, x 3
- Garlic, 1 teaspoon
- Portobello mushroom caps, 1 or 3 oz
- Cider vinegar, 0.25 cup
- Water, 1 cup
- Asparagus, 1lb
- Green peas, 0.5 cup
- Heavy cream, 2 tablespoons
- Basil, x 8 leaves
- Salt, 0.25 teaspoon
- Black pepper, 0.25 teaspoon

Method

- Melt 2 tablespoons of butter of a medium to high heat, once melted reduce to medium
- Add the scallions/spring onions and cook until wilted, for around 3 minutes
- Add the garlic and cook for half a minute
- Add the rest of the butter and the mushrooms, stir occasionally until the mushrooms are soft, for around 5 minutes
- Add the vinegar and cook for a further 2 minutes
- Pour the water into the pan
- Add the asparagus and bring to the boil
- Reduce the heat down to medium and simmer for 5 minutes
- Add the peas and cook for 2 minutes
- Add the heavy cream and simmer until the sauce thickens up, for about 2 minutes
- Transfer the mixture into a serving dish and stir in the basil

- Season with salt and pepper

Cauliflower with Red Pepper and Black Olives

Protein 2.9g, fat 6.7g, fiber 2.9g, calories 90, net carbs 4g
Serves 6

Ingredients

- Cauliflower, 1 x large head
- Roasted bell peppers, 4oz
- Pitted Kalamata olives, x 10
- Extra virgin olive oil, 2 tablespoons
- Parsley, 2 tablespoons

Method

- Cook the cauliflower and bring to the boil, usually for around 6-7 minutes – the cauliflower should be tender but firm
- Drain the cauliflower
- Mix in the bell pepper, olives, oil and the parsley
- Season with salt and pepper
- Serve

Chicken Pesto Salad

Protein 23.3g, fat 20.8g, fiber 0.8g, calories 296, net carbs 1.6g
Serves 4

Ingredients

- Onions (chopped), 1/3 cup
- Chicken breast (cooked and diced), 2 cups
- Celery, x 1 stalk
- Real mayonnaise, 1/3 cup
- Parsley, 2 tablespoons
- Pesto sauce, 2 tablespoons
- Salt, 0.25 teaspoon
- Black pepper, 1/8 teaspoon

Method

- Combine all ingredients together in a large bowl
- Serve straight away
- You can also add in cherry tomatoes as a garnish, however remember to add them into your carb count for the day

Afterword

And there you have it! You can now see how easy and delicious the Atkins Diet is, and it's not at all complicated. The recipes and food suggestions we have made are all super-healthy, packed with vitamins and minerals for overall health, but also have that added benefit of boosting weight loss, and allowing you to lead a healthier lifestyle for the rest of your days.

All you need to do is make sure that you don't go over your carb allowance per day, that you make sure you get enough protein, you drink enough water, and you add salt to your meals wherever applicable. Throw in some regular exercise and you will soon begin to reap the benefits of the Atkins Diet.

The fourth phase is really about the rest of your life, hence why we haven't given you a meal plan for that particular phase. This part is about flexibility and learning to make healthy choices over unhealthy ones. You can be a little less strict in this phase, i.e. you don't have to plan everything out quite as strictly as you did in the first phase or the second one, but it's important not to become complacent either.

If you have any concerns about starting the Atkins Diet, remember to discuss them with your doctor before you begin. It's also important to remember that the side effects we listed are only temporary, so it's really a case of gritting your teeth and working through them, to enable you to get to the green grass beyond that point! If, however, these side effects are severe or very prolonged, discuss with your doctor before you continue.

Now, it's time to head to the supermarket, stock up on those ingredients we have listed in each phase's shopping list, and get creating some of those delicious meals to enjoy as part of your journey towards a happier, healthier and slimmer future!

Good luck!

Copyright 2019 by Emilia Roberts - All rights reserved.

All rights Reserved. No part of this publication or the information in it may be quoted from or reproduced in any form by means such as printing, scanning, photocopying or otherwise without prior written permission of the copyright holder.

Disclaimer and Terms of Use: Effort has been made to ensure that the information in this book is accurate and complete, however, the author and the publisher do not warrant the accuracy of the information, text and graphics contained within the book due to the rapidly changing nature of science, research, known and unknown facts and internet. The Author and the publisher do not hold any responsibility for errors, omissions or contrary interpretation of the subject matter herein. This book is presented solely for motivational and informational purposes only.

Made in the USA
Middletown, DE
25 April 2019